Ubaid Amir
Yasmin Ansari

Anatomy and Physiology with Unani Review

Ubaid Amir
Yasmin Ansari

Anatomy and Physiology with Unani Review

LAP LAMBERT Academic Publishing

Cover image: www.ingimage.com

Publisher:
LAP LAMBERT Academic Publishing
is a trademark of
Dodo Books Indian Ocean Ltd. and OmniScriptum S.R.L publishing group

120 High Road, East Finchley, London, N2 9ED, United Kingdom
Str. Armeneasca 28/1, office 1, Chisinau MD-2012, Republic of Moldova, Europe
Managing Directors: Ieva Konstantinova, Victoria Ursu
info@omniscriptum.com

Printed at: see last page
ISBN: 978-620-8-43454-0

ANATOMY

Anatomy: the word anatomy is derived from a Greek word "Anatome" meaning to cut up. It is the study of structures that make up the body and how those structures relate with each other.

The study of anatomy includes many sub specialties. These are Microscopic anatomy, Gross anatomy, Developmental anatomy and Embryology etc.

Gross anatomy: Studies body structure with-out microscope. Systemic anatomy studies functional relationships of organs within a system whereas regional anatomy studies body part regionally. Both systemic and regional approaches may be used to study gross anatomy.

Microscopic anatomy (Histology): Requires the use of microscope to study tissues that form the various organs of the body.

Anatomical Position: Anatomical positions are universally accepted as the starting points for positional references to the body. In anatomical position the subject is standing erect and facing the observer, the feet are together, and the arms are hanging at the sides with the palms facing forward.

Organ: Is an integrated collection of two or more kinds of tissue that works together to perform specific function. For example: Liver, Stomach etc.

System: Is a group of organs that work together to perform major function. For example: Respiratory system contains several organs.

Organism level: The various organs of the body form the entire organism.

Term	*Meaning and Example*
Anterior (ventral)	Toward the front part of the body. The eye is anterior to the ears.
Posterior (dorsal)	Towards the back of the body. The ears are posterior to the nose
Medial	Towards the midline of the body. The nose is medial to the eyes.
Lateral	Away from the midline of the body. The eyes are lateral to the nose.
Superior (cranial)	Toward the head. The leg is supper to the foot.
Inferior (caudal)	Toward the feet. The foot is inferior to the leg.
Proximal Toward (nearer)	The trunk of the body or the attached end of a limb. The shoulder is proximal to the wrist.
Distal Away (farther)	From the trunk of the body or the attached end of a limb. The wrist is distal to the forearm.
Superficial	Nearer the surface of the body. The ribs are superficial to the heart.

Deep	Farther from the surface of the body. The heart is deeper to the ribs.
Peripheral	Away from the central axis of the body. Peripheral nerves radiate away from the brain and spinal cord.

Plane	*Meaning*
Sagittal plane	Divides the body into right and left half.
Mid sagittal plane	Divides body into equal left and right halves.
Para sagittal plane	Divides body into unequal left and right
Frontal plane	Divides the body into asymmetrical anterior and posterior sections.
Transverse plane	Divides the body into upper and lower body section.
Oblique plane	Divides the body obliquely into upper and lower section.

Adult Skeleton:

Axial Skeleton	*Appendicular skeleton*
Skull **Cranium 8** Parietal (2) Temporal (2) Frontal (1) Ethmoid (1) Sphenoid (1) Occipital (1)	**Upper extremities (64 bones)** Pectoral (shoulder) girdle 4 Clavicle (2) Scapula (2) **Wrist 16** Carpals (16)
Face 14 Maxillary (2) Zygomatic (molar) (2) Lacrimal (2) Nasal (2) Inferior nasal conchii (2) Palatine (2) Mandible (1) Vomer (1)	**Arms 2** Humerus (2) 4 Forearm Ulna (2) Radius (2) **Hand and fingers 38** Metacarpals (10) Phalanges (28)
Ossicles of ear 6: Malleus (hammer) (2) Incus (anvil) (2) Stapes (stirrup) (2) **Hyoid 1**	**Lower extremities (62 bones)** Pelvic girdle 2 (Fused ileum, ischium, pubis) **Thigh 4** Femur (2) Patella (2)
Vertebral column (26 bones) Cervical vertebrae 7 Thoracic vertebrae 12 Lumbar vertebrae 5 Sacrum (5 fused bones) 1 Coccyx (3- 5 fused bones) 1	**Leg 4** Tibia (2) Fibula (2)
Thorax (25bones)	**Ankle 14**

Ribs 24 Sternum 1	Tarsals (14)
Total axial bones (80)	**Foot and toes 38** Metatarsals (10) Phalanges (28)
	Total Appendicular bones 126

- The number of skull bones is sometimes listed as 22, when the Ossicles of the ears (6 bones) and the single hyoid bone is counted separately. Technically, the hyoid bone is not part of the skull.

DIAPHRAGMATIC OPENINGS

- Level of vena cava opening: **T8** (Pneumonic word vena cava contains 8 words so it can be related with T8).
- Level of oesophagus opening: **T10** (Pneumonic word oesophagus contains 10 words so it can be related with T10).
- Level of aorta Hiatus opening: **T12**. (Pneumonic word aorta Hiatus contains 12 words so it can be related with T12)
- Caval opening is through: Central part **(C-C)**
- Aortic opening is through: Osseo-aponeurotic opening **(not a true opening)**
- Oesophageal opening is through: Muscular part of diaphragm.
- Right phrenic nerve passes through: Vena caval opening (Right hand used for PV)
- Vagus nerve passes through: oesophageal opening. (Vagus 10th cranial nerve and oesophagus contains 10 words)
- Esophageal branch of left gastric artery passes through: Esophageal opening.
- Azygous vein passes through: **Aortic opening (AVA)**

ARTERIES

- Formed by union of 2 vertebral arteries: **Basilar Artery**.
- Inferior vesical artery is a branch of: Anterior division of internal iliac artery.
- Uterine Artery: is a branch of anterior division of internal iliac Artery.
- Inferior thyroid Artery: is a branch of Thyrocervical trunk.
- Ascending pharyngeal Artery: is a branch of: External carotid Artery.
- Internal pudendal Artery: is a branch of anterior division of **Internal iliac Artery.**
- Left gastro-epiploic Artery: is a branch of Splenic Artery.
- Splenic Artery: is a branch of Coeliac trunk.
- Cystic Artery: is a branch of Right hepatic Artery.
- Cilio-retinal Artery: is a branch of Choroidal Artery.
- Middle meningeal Artery: is a branch of Maxillary Artery.
- Anterior spinal Artery: is a branch of Vertebral Artery.
- Ophthalmic Artery: is a branch of Internal carotid Artery.
- Medially, superior thyroid artery is related to: External branch of superior laryngeal nerve.

EMBRYOLOGY

- Prochordal plate & primitive streak is seen on: **14th day**
- Oogonia & germ cell are derived from: **Yolk sac**
- 1st polar body is formed during: **Oogenesis.**
- 1st polar body is extruded: At the time of ovulation.
- Y chromosome is: **Acrocentric.**
- Blood cells and blood vessels are mesodermal in origin.
- Tongue muscles originate from myoblast of occiput somites.
- Sperms are stored in: **Epididymis.**
- Length of human sperm: **50-60 microns.**
- Number of chromosomes are reduced down to half in: **1st meiotic division.**
- In humans, implantation begins on the: **6th day after fertilization.**
- Initiation and maintenance of primitive streak is because of: **Nodal gene.**
- Primitive streak develops in which week: **3rd week.**
- Structure developed from cloaca: The cloaca develops into the rectum and upper 2/3 of the anal canal.
- Anomaly of pancreas in which the parts of the pancreas derived from the dorsal & ventral buds fail to fuse with each other: **Divided pancreas.**

FETAL STRUCTURES & ADULT REMNANTS:

- Meckel's divertculum: Remnant of **vitelline duct.**
- Ligamentum venosum: Remnant of **ductus venosus.**
- Ligamentum arteriosum: Remnant of **ductus arteriosus.**
- Median umbilical ligament: Remnant of **urachus.**
- Medial umbilical ligaments: Remnant of **2 umbilical arteries.**

DERIVATIVES OF GERMS LAYERS:

- **Mesodermal in origin:** Kidney, All Muscles (EXCEPT musculature of iris), Bone etc.
- **Trigone of bladder:** Mesoderm.
- **Somites:** Paraxial mesoderm.
- **Epithelial lining of biliary tract:** Endoderm.
- **Tympanic membrane:** All the 3 germ layers.

- **Derivatives of neural crest:**
- Neurons of Dorsal root, Sensory & Autonomic/ sympathetic ganglia, Schwann cells, Melanocytes, Mesenchyme of dental papillae etc.

EMBRYOLOGY OF GENITOURINARY SYSTEM

- Collecting duct develops from: **Ureteric bud.**
- Epithelium of ureter develops from: **Mesonephros.**
- Uterus/ appendix testes develops from: **Mullerian duct/ paramesonephric duct.**
- Ovary develops from: **Genital ridge.**
- Scrotum develops from: **Genital swelling.**
- Clitoris develops from: **Genital tubercle.**
- Penis develops from: **Genital Tubercle.**

POSITIONS OF THE TESTIS

- Iliac fossa: **3th months.**
- Deep inguinal ring: **4-6th months.**
- Pass through inguinal canal: **7th months.**
- Reach superficial inguinal ring: **8th months.**
- Reach scrotum: **8th months.**
- Bottom of scrotum: **9th months.**

PHARYNEGEAL ARCH DERIVATIVES

- Meckel's cartilage develops from: **1st pharyngeal arch.**
- Spheno-mandibular ligament develops from: **1st pharyngeal arch.**
- Stapes develops from**: 2nd pharyngeal arch.**
- Stylohyoid ligament develops from: **2nd pharyngeal arch.**
- Greater cornua of hyoid develops from: **3rd pharyngeal arch.**
- Posterior belly of digastric develops from: **2nd pharyngeal arch.**
- Anterior belly of digastric develops from: **1st pharyngeal arch.**
- Platysma develops from: **2nd pharyngeal arch.**

DERIVATIVES OF PHARYNGEAL POUCHES

- Palatine tonsil develops from: **2nd pharyngeal pouch.**
- Inferior parathyroid gland & thymus develops from: **3rd pharyngeal pouch.**

- Superior parathyroid gland & ultimobranchial body develops from: **4th pharyngeal pouch.**
- Parafollicular cells are derived from: **Ultimobranchial body.**

EPITHELIUM

- Mesothelium of pleura, peritoneum & pericardium is lined by: **Simple squamous epithelium.**
- Nasal cavity, nasal air sinuses, nasopharynx, larynx, trachea & bronchi are lined by: Ciliated pseudo-stratified columnar epithelium (EXCEPT vocal cords)
- True vocal cords, cornea, tonsil & vagina are lined by: Non keratinized stratified squamous epithelium.
- Epithelium with extra reserve of cell membrane: Transitional epithelium.
- Calyces, ureter, ureterovesical junction & urinary bladder have: Transitional epithelium.

HISTOLOGICAL FEATURES

- Brunner's gland is present in: **Duodenum.**
- Function of gap junctions: Exchange between cells.
- Gustatory system has: Sensory type of neuro-epithelium.
- Intercalated disc is present in: Cardiac muscle.
- Nucleus in cardiac muscle: **Central.**
- Reticuloendothelial cells of liver are: **Kupffer cells.**
- Space of Disse & space of Mall are seen in: **Liver.**
- Intrinsic factor (Castle) is secreted by: **Parietal/ oxyntic cells.**
- Chief/ peptic/ zymogen cells lines the: Body of the gland (secrete pepsinogen).
- Paneth cells (intestine) are rich in: **Rough ER.**
- Epiglottis is an example of: **Elastic cartilage.**

BRACHIAL PLEXUS

- Nerve arising from the trunks of brachial plexus: Suprascapular nerve, Subclavius nerve,
- Musculocutaneous nerve arises from: Lateral cord
- Subscapular nerve arises from: Posterior cord
- Erbs point is: Union of C5 & C6
- Erb's palsy involves: Upper trunk of brachial plexus

- Klumpke's paralysis is: Injury to lower trunk of brachial plexus

HAND

- Hypothenar area (medial third of palm) is supplied by: **Ulnar nerve**
- Palmar & dorsal interossei are supplied by: **Ulnar nerve**
- Adductor pollicis (adduction of thumb) is supplied by: **Ulnar nerve**
- Froment sign/ Book test is done for: **Ulnar nerve injury**
- Thenar eminence is supplied by: **Median nerve**
- Lunate dislocation may injure: **Median nerve**
- Ape thumb deformity is seen in: **Median nerve injury**

HIP & THIGH

- Nerve of medial/ adductor compartment of thigh: **Obturator nerve**
- Gluteus maximus is supplied by: **Inferior gluteal nerve**
- Gluteus minimus, G. medius & tensor fascia lata is supplied by: **Superior gluteal nerve**
- Action of sartorius & piriformis: Lateral rotation
- Superior & inferior gemelli action: Lateral rotation
- Abductors of the hip: Gluteus medius & gluteus minimus
- Function of ileofemoral ligament/ ligament of Bigelow: Prevents hyperextension at the hip
- Root value of pudendal nerve: **S2, S3, S4**
- Root value of obturator nerve: **L2, L3, L4**

KNEE

- Extensor of the knee joint: Quadricep femoris
- Posterior dislocation of femur is prevented by: Anterior cruciate ligament
- Posterior dislocation of the tibia is prevented by: Posterior cruciate ligament

ESOPHAGUS

- Esophagus pierces diaphragm at a distance of: 15 inches (from incisor)
- Length of esophagus: 25 cm
- Esophagus commences at: Lower end of cricoids
- Epithelium of esophagus: Stratified squamous non keratinized
- Most common site for oesophageal obstruction: Crico-oesophageal junction

HEART

- SA node, AV node & AV bundle is supplied by: Right coronary artery.
- Right coronary artery arises from: Anterior aortic cusp.
- Base of heart is formed by: **Both atrium.**
- Inferior surface of the heart is formed by: **Both ventricles.**
- Part of heart lying close to esophagus: **Left atrium.**
- Trabeculae carnea is present in: **Right ventricle.**
- Anterior wall of left ventricle is supplied by: Left anterior descending artery.
- In right dominance, posterior interventricular artery originates from: Right coronary artery.
- Middle cardiac vein follows: Posterior interventricular artery.
- SVC & IVC opens into: **Right atrium.**
- Coronary sinus drains into: Right atrium.

CRANIAL NERVES

- Artery crossing optic nerve: Ophthalmic artery.
- Cranial nerve having longest intracranial course: Trochlear
- Cranial nerve 3 & 4 have their nuclei in: Midbrain
- Cranial nerve 9, 10, 11, 12 have their nuclei in: Medulla
- Cranial nerve emerging from the dorsal aspect of brain: Trochlear.
- Muscles supplied by facial nerve: Platysma, Muscles of facial expression, Buccinator etc.
- Glands supplied by facial nerve: Submandibular, Lacrimal,Nasal glands
- Gustatory sensation to soft palate is carried by: **Facial nerve**
- Ganglion related to facial nerve: Pterygopalatine ganglion, Geniculate ganglion etc.
- Right hypoglossal nerve palsy will deviate the tongue to: Right side
- Arterial supply to facial nerve: Ascending pharyngeal artery
- All palatal muscles (except tensor palati) are supplied by: Cranial part of Accessory, nerve.
- Paralysis of 3, 4 & 6 cranial nerve indicates lesion of: Cavernous sinus (these nerve lies in lateral wall of cavernous sinus)
- Afferent pathway of corneal reflex: Trigeminal nerve (nasociliary branch of ophthalmic/ V1 division)

FORAMEN OF SKULL

- Contents of optic canal: Optic nerve & Ophthalmic artery
- Contents of foramen rotundum: Maxillary division of cranial nerve V
- Contents of foramen ovate: Mandibular division of cranial nerve V, Accessory meningeal artery etc.
- Contents of foramen spinosum: Middle meningeal artery,
- Meningeal branch of the mandibular nerve etc.
- Contents of foramen magnum: Accessory nerve, Vertebral & spinal arteries etc.
- Contents of jugular foramen: 9, 10 & 11 cranial nerves, Internal jugular vein, Inferior petrosal sinus.
- Contents of internal auditory meatus: 7 & 8 cranial nerve,
- Labyrinthine artery
- Content of Dorellos canal: Cranial nerve 6

LARYNX

- Cartilages of larynx: 3 paired & 3 unpaired.
- Sensory innervation above the level of vocal cords is by: Internal laryngeal nerve.
- Sensory innervation of larynx below the level of vocal cords: Recurrent laryngeal nerve.
- Nerve supply of cricothyroid: External laryngeal nerve.
- Abductor of vocal cords: Posterior crico-arytenoid.
- Tensor of vocal cords: Cricothyroid.

BRAIN

- Primary auditory area is in: Superior part of the temporal gyrus
- Primary visual area is in: Occipital lobe
- Loss of tactile localization & 2 point discrimination occurs in damage to: Somatosensory area 1
- Functions of limbic system: Emotions, Memory & Higher functions

LYMPAHTIC DRAINAGE

- Lymphatics drainage of testis: Para-aortic node
- Clitoris & glans Penis: Cloquet node/ Rossen mullers node
- Labium majus: Superficial inguinal node

- Testis: Pre-aortic & para-aortic nodes
- Tip of tongue: Submental nodes
- Spongiform urethra: Deep inguinal nodes
- Lymphatics are not present in: Brain, choroid, internal ear, cornea

VEINS

- Left gonadal vein drain into: Left renal vein.
- Great cerebral vein (of Galen) is formed by the union of: Internal cerebral veins.
- Great cerebral vein drains into: Straight sinus.
- Portal vein is formed by: Union of splenic vein & superior mesenteric vein (behind neck of pancreas).
- Normal portal pressure is: **5-10 mm Hg.**

STRUCTURE PASSING THROUGH THE FORAMEN

- Foramen Ovale: Mandibular nerve, Accessary meningeal nerve, Lesser petrosal nerve and Emissary vein. (Pneumonic MALE).
- Foramen Spinosum: Middle meningeal artery, emissary vein and nervus spinosus. (Pneumonic MEN).
- Foramen Lacerum: Meningeal branch of Ascending pharyngeal artery, emissary vein and other structure.
- Carotid canal: Internal carotid artery & venous and sympathetic plexus around it.
- Foramen rotundum: Maxillary nerve.

EXCEPTS' IN ANATOMY

- All intrinsic muscle of larynx are supplied by recurrent laryngeal nerve except: Cricothyroid **(external laryngeal nerve)**
- All muscles of tongue are supplied by hypoglossal nerve except: **Palatoglossus (pharyngeal plexus)**
- All muscles of pharynx are supplied by pharyngeal plexus except: **Stylopharyngeus (Glossopharyngeal nerve)**
- All muscles of the soft palate are supplied by pharyngeal plexus except: **Tensor palati (nerve to medial pterygoid)**

Quick Review

1. Superior & inferior radioulnar joints are an example of: Pivot joint.

2. Nerve supply of platysma: Facial nerve.

3. Salivary gland, NOT supplied by facial nerve: Parotid.

4. All palatal muscles are supplied by cranial accessory nerve through pharyngeal plexus except: Tensor veli palatini.

5. Azygos vein passes through Aortic hiatus.

6. Source of bleeding in extradural hemorrhage: Middle Meningeal artery.

7. Haversian canal is a histological feature of: Compact bone/ cortex.

8. Uterine artery is a branch of: Anterior division of Iliac artery.

9. 1st polar body is extruded at the time of: Ovulation.

10. Meckel's diverticulum is a remnant of: Vitello-intestinal duct.

11. Structure derived from all the three germ layers: Tympanic membrane/ ear drum.

12. Stapes develop from IInd pharyngeal arch.

13. Safety muscle of tongue: Genioglossus.

14. Taste sensation from anterior 2/3rd of tongue is carried by: Chorda tympani.

15. Epithelial lining of tonsil: Stratified squamous non-keratinized epithelium.

16. Peritoneal cavity is lined by: Simple squamous epithelium.

17. Intercalated disc is a histological feature of: Cardiac muscle.

18. Erb's point is: C5, C6.

19. Injury to lower trunk of brachial plexus is known as: Klumpke's palsy.

20. Adductor pollicis is supplied by: Ulnar nerve.

21. Teres minor & deltoid muscle are supplied by: Axillary nerve.

22. Nerve supply of gluteus maximus: Inferior gluteal nerve.

23. Ligament preventing hyperextension at the hip joint: Iliofemoral ligament/ Ligament of Bigelow.

24. Inversion & eversion occurs at Subtalar joint.

25. Joint between epiphysis & diaphysis is: Primary cartilaginous.

26. Vessels in umbilical cord:2 arteries & 1 vein (right vein disappears, left vein is LEFT).

27. Ligamentum arteriosum is derived from: Ductus arteriosus.

28. Artery present in anatomical snuff box: Radial artery.

29. Sperm are stored in: Epididymis.

30. Hassal's corpuscles is seen in: Thymus.

31. Peyer's patches are present in: Ileum.

32. Nerve supply to hypothenar muscle is from: Ulnar nerve.

33. Nerve passing deep to flexor retinaculum at wrist: Median nerve.

34. Nerve related to spiral groove of humerus: Radial nerve.

35. Azygos veins drain into: Superior Vena Cava.

36. Housemaid's knee is inflammation of Prepatellar bursa.

37. Superficial inguinal ring is a defect in the: External oblique aponeurosis.

38. Left testicular vein drains into: Left renal vein.

39. Left gastro-epiploic artery is a branch of: Splenic artery.

40. MC position of appendix: Retrocaecal.

41. Nasolacrimal duct opens into inferior meatus.

42. Parasympathetic secretomotor fibres to submandibular gland is through: Facial nerve.

43. Opening of parotid duct: opposite upper 2nd molar.

44. Abductor of vocal cord: Posterior cricoarytenoid.

45. In adults spinal cord ends at the lower border of L1 vertebra (in children, it is at lower border of L3).

46. Muscle supplied by spinal part of accessory nerve: Sternocleidomastid & trapezius muscle.

47. Unlocking of knee is done by: Popliteus.

48. Type of cartilage in auricle of ear: Elastic.

49. Nerve supply of superior oblique muscle: Trochlear.

50. Muscle producing abduction, intorsion & depression of eyeball: Superior Oblique.

51. Space of Disse seen in: Liver

52. Types of the epiphysis: pressure epiphysis, traction epiphysis, atavistic epiphysis and aberrant epiphysis.

53. Types of the joints: Fibrous joints, cartilaginous joints and synovial joints.

54. Bones develop through a process known as Ossification.

55. Bone in embryo develops in two ways: Intra-membranous ossification and Endochondrial Ossification.

56. Blood vessels present in the bone but not found in the cartilage.

57. Fungiform papillae found in the dorsum of the tongue.

58. Foliate papillae located in the lateral margin of the tongue.

59. Taste buds are present in tongue, palate, epiglottis, larynx, and esophagus.

Some Important Negative Points

- Alar ligament not present in TM Joint.
- Vitelline does not form the SVC.
- Spinal nerve is not supplied by Thoraco-acromial Artery.
- Breast is not supply by costoclavicular artery.
- Uterus does not drain into deep inguinal nodes.

- Fold of the gastrointestinal which are not permanent Rugae.
- Not a branch of axillary artery Dorsal scapular artery.
- Superior gluteal nerve does not supply to gluteus maximus.
- Ovary is not a content of the broad ligament.
- Femoral artery does not bound in the femoral ring.
- Femoral nerve does not seen in the femoral sheath.
- Root of the penis not a content of deep perineal pouch.
- Internal urethral sphincter does not a sphincter of vagina.
- Ligamentum teres not a derivatives of the septum transversum.

Easy to learn

Pneumonic:

- **Bowel components:**

  "Dow Jones Industrial Average Closing Stock Report"

  1. Duodenum
  2. Jejunum
  3. Ileum
  4. Appendix
  5. Colon
  6. Sigmoid
  7. Rectum

- **Duodenum: lengths of parts**

  "Counting 1 to 4 but staggered"

  1. 1st part: 2 inches
  2. 2nd part: 3 inches
  3. 3rd part: 4 inches
  4. 4th part: 1 inch.

- **Meckel's diverticulum details:**

  "**di-**" means "**two**", so diverticulum is the thing with all the **twos**

1. 2 inches long.
2. 2 feet from end of ileum.
3. 2 times more common in men.

4. 2% occurrence in population.
5. 2 types of tissues may be present.

- **Aorta vs. vena cava: right vs. left:**

1. Aorta and right each have 5 letters, so aorta is on the right.
2. Vena and cava and left each have 4 letters, so vena cava is on the left.

- **Aortic arch: major branch order:**

"Know your ABC'S":

1. Aortic arch gives rise to:
2. Brachiocephalic trunk
3. left Common Carotid
4. left Subclavian

- **Atrioventricular valves:**

"<u>LAB</u> <u>RAT</u>":

1. Left Atrium: Bicuspid.
2. Right Atrium: Tricuspid.

- **Axillary artery branches:**

"Screw The Lawyer Save A Patient"

"<u>S</u>ome <u>T</u>imes <u>L</u>ife <u>S</u>eems <u>A</u> <u>P</u>ain"

1. Superior thoracic
2. Thoracoacromiol
3. Lateral thoracic
4. Subscapular
5. Anterior circumflex humeral
6. Posterior circumflex humeral

- **Brachial artery: recurrent and collateral branches.**

"<u>I</u> <u>A</u>m <u>P</u>retty <u>S</u>exy"

1. **I**nferior ulnar collateral artery goes with **A**nterior ulnar recurrent artery.
2. **P**osterior ulnar recurrent artery goes with **S**uperior ulnar collateral artery.

- **Carotid sheath contents**

"<u>I See</u> <u>10 CC</u>'s in the <u>IV</u>"

1. I See (I.C.) = Internal Carotid artery
2. 10 = CN 10 (Vagus nerve)
3. CC = Common Carotid artery
4. IV = Internal Jugular Vein

➢ **Cavernous sinus contents:**

O TOM CAT:

1. Occulomotor nerve (III)
2. Trochlear nerve (IV)
3. Ophthalmic nerve (V1)
4. Maxillary nerve (V2)
5. Carotid artery
6. Abducent nerve (VI)
7. T: Nothing.

➢ **Coelic trunk: branches:**

Left Hand Side (LHS):

1. Left gastric artery.
2. Hepatic artery.
3. Splenic artery.

➢ **Descending abdominal aorta branches from diaphragm to iliacs:**

"Prostitutes Cause Sagging Swollen Red Testicles [in men] Living In Sin"

1. Phrenic [inferior]
2. Celiac
3. Superior mesenteric
4. Suprarenal [middle]
5. Renal
6. Testicular ["in men" only]
7. Lumbars
8. Inferior mesenteric
9. Sacral

➢ **External carotid artery branches:**

"Some Anatomists Like F*#king, Others Prefer S & M"

1. Superior thyroid

2. Ascending pharyngeal
3. Lingual
4. Facial
5. Occipital
6. Posterior auricular
7. Superficial temporal
8. Maxillary

- **Femoral triangle: arrangement of contents:**

NAVEL:

From lateral hip towards medial navel.

1. Nerve (directly behind sheath)
2. Artery (within sheath)
3. Vein (within sheath)
4. Empty space (between vein and lymph)
5. Lymphatics (with deep inguinal node).

- **Heart valve sequence:**

"Try Pulling My Aorta"

1. **T**ricuspid
2. **P**ulmonary
3. **M**itral
4. **A**orta

- **Inferior vena cava tributaries:**

"I Like To Rise So High"

1. Iliac
2. Lumbar
3. Testicular
4. Renal
5. Suprarenal
6. Hepatic vein.

- **Internal jugular vein: tributaries**

"Medical Schools Let Confident People In"

From inferior to superior:

1. Middle thyroid
2. Superior thyroid
3. Lingual
4. Common facial
5. Pharyngeal
6. Inferior petrosal sinus

- **Thoracic cage: relations to the important venous structures:**

Behind the sternoclavicular joints:

the brachiocephalic veins begin.

1. Behind the 1st costal cartilage on the right the superior vena cava begins.
2. Behind the 2nd costal cartilage on the right the azygos vein ends.
3. Behind the 3rd costal cartilage on the right the superior vena cava ends.

- **Thoracoacromial artery branches:**

ABCD:

1. Acromial
2. Breast (pectoral)
3. Clavicular
4. Deltoid.

- **Scalp layers:**

<u>SCALP</u>:

From superficial to deep:

1. **S**kin
2. **C**onnective tissue
3. **A**poneurosis
4. **L**oose areolar tissue
5. **P**ericranium

- **Spleen: dimensions, weight, surface anatomy:**

"1,3,5,7,9,11"

1. Spleen dimensions are 1 inch x 3 inches x 5 inches.
2. Weight is 7 ounces.
3. It underlies ribs 9 through 11.

➢ **Thoracic duct: relation to azygous vein and esophagus:**

"The duck between 2 gooses"

1. Thoracic duct (duck) is between 2 gooses, azygous and esophagus.

➢ **Abdominal muscles:**

"Spare TIRE around their abdomen"

1. Transversus abdominis
2. Internal abdominal oblique
3. Rectus abdominis
4. External abdominal oblique

➢ **Bicipital groove: attachments of muscles near it.**

"The lady between two majors"

1. Teres major attaches to medial lip of groove.
2. Pectoralis major to lateral lip of groove.
3. Latissimus (Lady) is on floor of groove, between the 2 majors.

➢ **Elbow: muscles that flex it.**

Three B's Bend the elBow:

1. Brachialis
2. Biceps
3. Brachioradialis.

➢ **Elbow: which side has common flexor origin.**

1. **FM** (as in FM Radio):
2. **F**lexor **M**edial, so Common Flexor Origin is on the medial side.

➢ **Erector spinae muscles:**

"I Love South Indians"

From lateral to medial:

1. Iliocostalis
2. Longissimus
3. Spinalis

➢ **Eye rotation by oblique muscles:**

"I Love S&M"

1. Inferior oblique: Lateral eye rotation.
2. Superior oblique: Medial eye rotation.

➢ **Intrinsic muscles of hand (palmar surface):**

"A OF A OF A"

Thenar, lateral to medial:

1. **A**bductor pollicis longus
2. **O**pponens pollicis
3. **F**lexor pollicis brevis
4. **A**dductor pollicis.

Hypothenar, lateral to medial:

1. **O**pponens digiti minimi
2. **F**lexor digiti minimi
3. **A**bductor digiti minimi

➢ **Lumbricals action:**

Lumbrical action is to hold a pea, that is to flex the metacarpophalangeal joint and extend the interphalangeal joints.

➢ **Muscles: potentially absent ones:**

Muscles which may be absent but may be important:

➢ **5 P's:**

1. **P**almaris longus [upper limb]
2. **P**lantaris [lower limb]
3. **P**eroneus tertius [lower limb]
4. **P**yramidalis [anterior abdominal wall]
5. **P**soas minor [posterior abdominal wall]

➢ **Rotator cuff muscles:**

"The SITS muscles"

Clockwise from top:

1. Supraspinatus
2. Infraspinatus
3. Teres minor
4. Subscapularis

- **Serratus anterior: innervation.**

"SALT"

1. Serratus Anterior = Long Thoracic.
2. Soleus vs. gastrocnemius muscle function.

"Stand on your Soles. Explosive gas"

1. You stand on soles of your shoes, so **Soleus** is for **posture**.
2. Gasoline is explosive, so **Gastrocnemius** is for **explosive** movement.

- **Supination vs. pronation:**

1. **"SOUPination"** Supination is to turn your arm palm up, as if you are holding a bowl of soup.
2. **"POUR-nation"** Pronation is to turn your arm with the palm down, as if you are pouring out whatever is your bowl.

- **Bell's palsy: symptoms.**

BELL'S Palsy:

1. Blink reflex abnormal
2. Earache
3. Lacrimation [deficient, excess]
4. Loss of taste
5. Sudden onset
6. Palsy of VII nerve muscles.

- **Brachial plexus subunits:**

"Randy Travis Drinks Cold Beer"

1. Roots
2. Trunks
3. Divisions
4. Cords
5. Branches

- **Brachial plexus: branches of posterior cord:**

STAR:

1. Subscapular [upper and lower]
2. Thoracodorsal

3. Axillary
4. Radial

➢ **Buttock quadrant safest for needle insertion:**

"Shut up and butt out"

The **Upper Ou**ter quadrant of the **Butt**ock safely avoids hitting sciatic nerve.

➢ **Carpal tunnel syndrome causes:**

MEDIAN TRAP:

1. **M**yxoedema
2. **E**dema premenstrually
3. **D**iabetes
4. **I**diopathic
5. **A**gromegaly
6. **N**eoplasm
7. **T**rauma
8. **R**heumatoid arthritis
9. **A**myloidosis
10. **P**regnancy

➢ **Cervical plexus: arrangement of the important nerves:**

"GLAST"

4 compass points: clockwise from north on the right side of neck.

1. **G**reat auricular
2. **L**esser occipital
3. **A**ccessory nerve pops out between L and S
4. **S**upraclavicular
5. **T**ransverse cervical

➢ **Deep tendon reflexes: root supply:**

1. **One, two**-- buckle my shoe.
2. **Three, four**-- kick the door.
3. **Five, six**-- pick up sticks.
4. **Seven, eight**-- shut the gate.
   - **S1,2** = ankle jerk
   - **L3,4** = knee jerk

- **C5,6** = biceps and brachioradialis
- **C7,8** = triceps

➢ **Diaphragm innervation:**

"3, 4, 5 keeps the diaphragm alive"

Diaphragm innervation is cervical roots 3, 4, and 5.

➢ **Extraocular muscles cranial nerve innervation:**

"LR6SO4 rest 3"

1. Lateral Rectus is 6th cranial nerve
2. Superior Oblique is 4th cranial nerve
3. Rest muscles are 3rd cranial nerve.

➢ **Facial nerve: branches after Stylomastoid foramen:**

"Ten Zulus Buggered My Cat (Painfully)"

From superior to inferior:

1. **T**emporal branch
2. **Z**ygomatic branch
3. **B**uccal branch
4. **M**andibular branch
5. **C**ervical branch (Posterior auricular nerve).

➢ **Lumbar plexus:**

"I, I Get Laid On Fridays"

1. **I**liohypogastric [L1]
2. **I**lioinguinal [L1]
3. **G**enitofemoral [L1, L2]
4. **L**ateral femoral cutaneous [L2, L3]
5. **O**btruator [L2, L3, L4]
6. **F**emoral [L2, L3, L4]

➢ **Lumbar plexus roots:**

"2 from 1, 2 from 2, 2 from 3"

1. 2 nerves from 1 root: **I**lioinguinal (L1), Iliohypogastric (L1).
2. 2 nerves from 2 roots: **G**enitofemoral (L1,L2), Lateral Femoral (L2,L3).
3. 2 nerves from 3 roots: **O**bturator (L2,L3,L4), Femoral (L2,L3,L4).

- **Median nerve: hand muscles innervated:**

"The LOAF muscles"

1. **L**umbricals 1 and 2
2. **O**pponens pollicis
3. **A**bductor pollicis brevis
4. **F**lexor pollicis brevis.

- **Median nerve: recognizing it in an opened axilla:**

The Median nerve is the Middle of a giant capital "M" formed by the musculocutaneous and ulnar nerves.

- **Radial nerve: muscles supplied (simplified):**

"BEST muscles"

1. **B**rachioradialis
2. **E**xtensors
3. **S**upinator
4. **T**riceps

- **Scalp: nerve supply:**

"GLASS"

1. **G**reater occipital/ Greater auricular
2. **L**esser occipital
3. **A**uriculotemporal
4. **S**upratrochlear
5. **S**upraorbital

- **Spinal cord: length in vertebral column:**

"SCULL"

Spinal Cord Unti L2 (LL).

- **Thigh: innervation by compartment:**

"MAP OF Sciatic"

1. **M**edial compartment: **O**bturator.
2. **A**nterior compartment: **F**emoral
3. **P**osterior compartment: Sciatica

- **Trigeminal nerve: where branches exit skull:**

"Standing Room Only"

1. **S**uperior orbital fissure is V1
2. Foramen **R**otundum is V2
3. Foramen **O**vale is V3

- **V3 (Third branch of the trigeminal) innervated muscles (branchial arch 1 derivatives):**

"M.D. My TV"

1. **M**astication [masseter, temporalis, pterygoids]
2. **D**igastric [anterior belly]
3. **M**ylohyoid
4. **T**ensor Tympani
5. **T**ensor Veli palatini.

- **V3: sensory branches:**

"Buccaneers Are Inferior Linguists"

1. **B**uccal
2. **A**uriculotemporal
3. **I**nferior alveolar
4. **L**ingual.

- **Vagus nerve: path into thorax:**

"I Left my Aunt in Vegas"

Left Vagus nerve goes **A**nterior descending into the thorax.

- **Cubital fossa contents:**

"Really Need Booze To Be At My Nicest"

From lateral to medial:

1. **R**adial Nerve
2. **B**iceps Tendon
3. **B**rachial Artery
4. **M**edian Nerve

- **Hand: nerve lesions:**

"DR CUMA"

1. **D**rop=Radial nerve
2. **C**law=Ulnar nerve
3. **M**edian nerve=Ape hand (or Apostol [preacher] hand).

PHYSIOLOGY

BODY FLUIDS

- Water constitutes about: 60% of entire body weight
- Sodium, chloride & bicarbonate ions are predominant found in: Extracellular fluid
- Intracellular fluid is rich in concentration of: Potassium
- Endolymph is rich in: Potassium.
- Measurement of total body water: Tritrated water, deuterium oxide (D_2O)
- Measurement of ECF: Inulin, mannitol etc.
- Measurement of plasma volume: Evans blue, radio labelled albumin.
- Normal anion gap (cations - anions): 10-12 mmol/ L.

NERVE & MUSCLE PHYSIOLOGY

- RMP is due to: Potassium ions.
- RMP of nerve fibre is: -70 Mv.
- RMP is close to iso-electric potential of: Chloride ions.
- At synapse, nerve impulse flow is: Unidirectional.
- Band which narrows during contraction: H-band.
- Active sites of actin are covered by: Tropomyosin.
- Essential for smooth muscle contraction: Cellular calcium.
- Order of susceptibility of nerve fibers to pressure: Type A > type B > type c.

CVS PHYSIOLOGY

- Resistance vessel: Artery/ arteriole.
- Exchange vessel: Capillaries (maximum surface area).
- Capacitance vessel: Vein.
- BP is calculated as: Cardiac output X peripheral resistance.
- Small cuff, thicken walled vessels & obesity will give a: High B.P
- Ventricular end diastolic volume: Volume of blood in ventricular cavity at the end of atrial contraction (120ml): determines preload
- Ejection fraction: Ratio of stroke volume to end diastolic volume (SD/ EDV): 50-70%
- Stroke volume: Volume of blood ejected with each heart beat (CO/ HR): 70-80 ml
- Cardiac index: Cardiac output/ Body surface area: 3.2 is the normal value.
- SA Node innervates with right vagus nerve.
- AV node innervates with left vagus nerve.
- Conduction rate of SA node is 0.05

- Conduction rate of AV node is 0.05
- Conduction rate of atrial pathways is 1.
- Conduction rate of budle of his is 1.
- Conduction rate of purkinje fibre is 4 (which is fastest).
- Conduction rate of ventricular muscle is 1.

ELECTROCARDIOGRAM

- Axis of lead I is 0 degree.
- Axis of lead II is + 60 degree.
- Axis of lead III is + 120 degree.
- The normal direction of the mean QRS vector is generally in between 30 degree to 110 degree.
- Duration of one cardiac cycle is 0.8 second.
- Duration of the ventricular systole is 0.3 second.
- Duration of the ventricular diastole is 0.5 second.
- Duration of the atrial systole is 0.1 second.
- Duration of atrial diastole is 0.7 second.
- QRS complex is due to: Ventricular depolarization
- Duration of QRS complex: 0.08 - 0.10 sec
- 3rd heart sound is hear during: Ventricular filling phase
- 'Y' wave in JVP is due to: Opening of AV valve & emptying of blood into ventricle.

Tissue	*Depolarization due to*
Nerve	Na^+ influx through voltage gated sodium channels.
Skeletal muscle	Na^+ influx through voltage gated sodium channels.
Smooth muscle	Ca^{2+} influx
SA Node	Ca^{2+} influx
Ventricular muscle	Na^+ influx
Inner hair cell of the Cochlea	K^+ influx

Nerve fiber classification:

Fibre type	*Functions*	**Fibre diameter**	**Conduction**
Alpha	Proprioception, somatic motor	12-20	70-120
Beta	High discrimination touch (fine touch), vibration, deep pressure.	5-12	30-70
Gamma	Motor to muscle spindles	3-6	15-30
Delta	Fast pain, temperature (Cold) touch	2-5	12-30
Dorsal root	Slow pain, temperature, crude touch, pressure, itch, tickle, some reflex responses.	0.4-1.2	0.5-2
Sympathetic	Postganglionic sympathetic	0.3-1.3	0.7-2.3

Vessels:

Vessels	*Features*
Wind kessel vessels	Ex: aorta, major arteries, have a lot of elastic tissue that show elastic recoil (wind kessel effect), when stretched.

Resistance vessels	Arterioles have some elastic tissue: have lot of smooth muscle (have the maximum wall thickness to lumen ratio).
Precapillary sphincter	No innervation, respond to local metabolites.
Exchange vessels	Capillaries, no innervation, Controlled by precapillary sphincter.
Capacitance vessels	Have some innervation (Vena cava have minimum thickness to lumen ratio).
Shunt vessels	Form arterio-venous anastomoses. They have thick muscular wall very richly innervated fingertips, earlobes etc.

- First 14 generations form the conduction zone (Consisting to bronchi, bronchioles and terminal bronchioles as 14th generations known as terminal bronchioles.
- 23 generation is alveoli.
- 15th to 18th generations are respiratory bronchioles.
- 19th to 22nd generations are alveolar ducts.
- Volume of the alveolar region is about 2.5 litre to 3.0
- Presence of cilia, smooth muscle, glands, cartilage in the air passage.
- Cillia present in the generations 0-11 absent in bronchioles.
- Glands present in only trachea and bronchi.
- Smooth muscle maximum in terminal bronchiole.
- Secretory surfactant is type II (Also known as granular pneumocytes).
- Normal value of the anatomical dead space is 150 ml.
- Factor affecting the diffusion capacity are area of the membrane, solubility of the gas, molecular weight of the gas, thickness of the membrane.
- The affinity of Hb for carbon monoxide is 210 times that for O^2.
- Less Hb is available for carrying O^2
- Factors affecting the respiratory centre are (chemical e.x carbon dioxide, oxygen, hydrogen) and (Non-chemical vagal afferents from airways/lungs, pons, limbic system, proprioceptors and baroreceptors.
- CO2 is primarily transported in arterial blood as: Bicarbonate
- During inspiration, intrapleural pressure becomes: More negative
- Total lung capacity: Volume of air contained in the lung at the end of maximal inspiration; 6 L (male); 4.7 L(female)
- Total lung capacity depends upon: Lung compliance
- Tidal volume: Amount of air breathed in or out during normal breathing; 500 ml (male); 390 ml (female).
- At the apex of lung: V (ventilation) > Q (perfusion) [wasted ventilation]
- Volume of lung at the end of quite expiration, which can be expired with maximal effect: Expiratory reserve volume
- Minute alveolar ventilation is: 3.5 - 4.5 L
- Response to high altitude:
  - Increased ventilation (earliest),
  - Increased response to carotid bodies,

- o Respiratory alkalosis etc.
- ➢ Pulmonary surfactant is secreted by: Type II pneumocytes
- ➢ Surfactant is: Dipalmitoyl lecithin
- ➢ Surfactant production is accelerated by: Glucocorticoids
- ➢ Respiratory distress syndrome is due to: Deficiency of surfactant
- ➢ Chloride shift: Bicarbonate diffuses into plasma & same quantity of chloride diffuses into RBC in venous circulation
- ➢ Pneumotaxic centre is present in: Pons (dorsal)
- ➢ Shape of oxygen hemoglobin dissociation curve: Sigmoid
- ➢ Decrease in temperature shifts the curve to: Left
- ➢ Increase in affinity of oxygen for hemoglobin shift the curve to: Left
- ➢ Increased pCO2 shift the curve to: Right
- ➢ Sickle cell hemoglobin presence shift the curve to: Right
- ➢ Respiratory distress syndrome shift the curve to: Right
- ➢ 2,3 DPG (increased in anemia) shift the curve to: Right
- ➢ MC type of hypoxia: Hypoxic hypoxia
- ➢ Hypoxia is defined as: Low pO2

EXCRETORY SYSTEM

- ➢ Action of renin: Converts angiotensinogen to angiotensin I
- ➢ Factors stimulating renin secretion:
- o Low B.P
- o Hyponatremia
- ➢ Major part of glomerular filtrate is absorbed in: PCT.
- ➢ Substances completely reabsorbed in PCT:
- o Glucose
- o Bicarbonate
- o Water
- ➢ In presence of vasopressin, maximum reabsorption of water takes place in: PCT (even in absence of
- o Vasopressin, maximum reabsorption of water takes place in PCT)
- ➢ Substances partially reabsorbed in PCT:
- o Sodium,
- o Potassium,
- o Chloride

- Glucose transport occurs with: Sodium
- Macula densa is: Epithelial lining of distal tubule
- Tubuloglomerular feedback is mediated by sensing: Sodium chloride in densa
- Loop of Henle does not handle: Urea
- Filtration fraction is calculated as: GFR/ RPF; 20%

GASTROINTESTINAL TRACT

- Site of absorption of iron: Duodenum
- Intrinsic factor is secreted by: Oxyntic/ parietal cells
- HCl is secreted by: Oxyntic/ parietal cells
- Gastrin is secreted by: G cells of stomach, duodenum etc.
- Action of gastrin:
  - Stimulates secretion of gastric juice,
  - Increases gastric motility etc.
- Action of secretin:
  - Stimulates secretion of watery, alkaline & pancreatic secretions, Inhibit gastric secretion,
  - Causes contraction of pyloric sphincter,
- Most potent stimulator of secretion of secretin is: Acidic chyme
- Action of cholecystokinin: Stimulates contraction of gallbladder
- CCK-PZ secretion is stimulated by: Proteins
- Gastric secretion is stimulated by:
  - Gastrin,
  - Histamine etc.
- Gastric phase of gastric secretion is mediated by: Hormones
- Intestinal motility is stimulated by:
  - Distension,
  - Acetylcholine etc.
- Fat is maximally absorbed in: Jejunum
- Calcium is maximally absorbed in: proximal intestine
- Electrolytes are absorbed in: Colon
- Effect of dietary fibres (e.g. pectin):
  - Increases bulk of stool,
  - Increases metabolism or sugar in GIT
- Largest reserve of energy in body: Fat
- Gastric lipase helps in digestion of: Fats

- Indicator of malabsorption: Fat in stool (> 6 gms/ day)

ENDOCRINOLOGY

- Insulin increases:
  - Glycogen synthesis,
  - Fat synthesis,
  - Protein synthesis etc.
- Insulin is a: Hypoglycemic hormone
- Insulin is secreted by: Beta cells of pancreas
- In fetus, secretion of insulin begins by: 3 months
- Insulin secretion is inhibited by: Epinephrine
- Delta cells of pancreas secrete: Somatostatin
- Hormones acting on intracellular nuclear receptors:
  - Steroids
  - Thyroid hormones
  - Vitamin-D etc.
- cAMP mediates action of:
  - ADH
  - PTH etc.
- cGMP mediates action of: NO (cellular signaling molecule)
- Insulin acts through: Tyrosine kinase activity
- Hormones belonging to steroid receptor family:
- Vitamin D3,
- Thyroid
- Effect of parathormone:
  - Stimulates osteoclastic activity,
  - Augments absorption of calcium from the gut
- Effect of calcitonin:

o Opposite to that of PTH,

o Lowers serum calcium,

o Acts by decreasing osteoclasis (bone resorption)

- Active form of calcium: Ionized form
- RMP of nerve fibre is: -70 Mv
- RMP of nerve fibre is: -70 Mv
- A decrease in concentration of free calcium ions in plasma results in:

o Increased neuromuscular irritability & tetani,

o Chvostek's sign etc.

- ECG finding of hypocalcemia: Lengthening of the QT interval
- ACTH & TSH are secreted by: Anterior pituitary gland
- Vasopressin & oxytocin are released by: Posterior pituitary gland

REPRODUCTIVE SYSTEM

- Functions of LH:

o Stimulates ovulation,

o Maintains corpus luteum

- FSH receptors are present in: Granulosa cells
- Hormonal status in menopause:

o Decreased estrogen,

o Raised FSH & LH

- Spermatozoa acquire motility in: Epididymis
- Capacitation occurs in: Female genital tract
- In female genital tract, sperm don't survive more than: 48 hours
- Testosterone is produced from: Pregnanolone
- Testosterone is produced by: Leydig cells
- Blood testis barrier is formed by: Sertoli cells
- Inhibin is secreted by: Sertoli cells
- Most useful physiologic marker of thyroid hormone action: TSH
- Hormones increased in stressful conditions:

o Adrenaline,

o Vasopressin,

o Cortisol,

o Glucagon,

- Insulin is NOT increased in stressful conditions
- Melatonin is a: Pineal hormone
- In darkness: Activity of serotonin-N-acetyl transferase is increased

NERVOUS SYSTEM

- Theta waves (4-7 Hz) are seen in: Hippocampus
- Delta waves (3-5 Hz) are seen in: Deep sleep

- Nightmares are seen in: REM sleep
- HelmHoltz theory (of colour vision): There are 3 kinds of cones in retina, corresponding to 3 colour's
- Protanomoly is: Defect in red cones
- Visible range of electromagnetic spectrum of human eye: 370-740 nm
- Function of amacrine cells: Regulates relative color & luminosity of photoreceptive input under changing light
- Most sensitive (pathway) for stimulus of colour contrast: Parvocellular pathway (from lateral geniculate body to visual cortex)
- Blobs of visual cortex are associated with: Colour processing
- Function of pacinian corpuscles: Senses rapidly adapting touch, pressure & vibration
- Region of CNS, which degenerate in Huntington's disease (GABAergic neurons): Caudate nucleus Cingulate gyri amygdaloid nucleus are part of: Limbic system
- Wernickes aphasia is: Impaired comprehension of spoken & written language
- Broacas aphasia is concerned with: Word formation
- Broacaa area is present in: Inferior frontal gyrus
- Nuclei of hypothalamus controlling thirst & water balance: Supraoptic nucleus
- Nuclei of hypothalamus controlling circadian rhythm: Suprachiasmatic nucleus
- Nuclei of hypothalamus controlling shivering: Posterolateral hypothalamus
- Class III Amino acids are GABA, Glycine, Glutamate etc.
- Hypothalamic releasing hormones are TRH, LH-RH, GH-IH.
- **Effect on the synaptic transmission:**
- Alkalosis: Increases synaptic transmission.
- Acidosis: Decrease synaptic transmission (Diabetic acidosis/uremic acidosis) etc.
- Hypoxia: Decrease excitability.
- Fatigue may occur due to exhustion.
- Parts of the thalamus are Epithalamus, Ventral thalamus, Dorsal thalamus etc.
- Medial geniculate body concerned with hearing. (**M**usic is hear)
- Lateral geniculate body concerned with vision.
- Ventro-posterior lateral and ventro-posterior medial (ventrobasal group of the nuclei).
- Thalamus is one of the best relay station for all types of the sensory functions.
- Also a crude centre for pre-ception of sensations.
- Role of synchronization of EEG.
- Functions of hypothalamus:

o Food intake,

o Hypophyseal control.

o Non shivering thermogenesis (because of noradrenaline; mediated by beta 3 receptors)

- Hormone important for cold adaptation: Thyroxine (piloerection is NOT significant)
- Main excitatory neurotransmitter in CNS is: Glutamate
- Functions of cerebellum:

o Coordinates & smoothens the action of different muscle groups,

o Producing smooth & accurate movements

- Intention tremors are seen in: Lesions of cerebellum
- Function of basal nuclei/ basal ganglia: Planning & programming of movements
- Caudate nucleus & lentiform nuclei (corpus striatum) are a part of: Basal ganglia

Quick Review

- Sperms mature inside the: Epididymis
- Vitamin-K dependent clotting factors: 2, 7, 9 10
- FSH is secreted by: **Anterior pituitary**
- Oxytocin is synthesized in: **Hypothalamus**
- Milk let down reflex is controlled by: **Oxytocin**
- Resting membrane potential is due to: Potassium ions
- Function of muscle spindle: Detects muscle tension
- Function of basal ganglia: Programming of muscle movements
- Intention tremors are seen in lesions of: Cerebellar lesions
- Main excitatory neurotransmitter in CNS: Glutamate
- Hormone important for cold adaptation: Thyroxine
- Hypothalamic nuclei controlling thirst & water balance: Supraoptic
- Broaca area is present in: Inferior frontal gyrus
- Impaired comprehension of spoken & written language is known as: Wernickes aphasia
- Nightmares are seen in: REM sleep
- Most useful physiologic marker of thyroid hormone action: TSH
- Blood testes barrier is formed by: Sertoli cells
- Testosterone is produced by: Leydig cells
- Capacitation occurs in: Female genital tract/ uterus
- Sperms acquire motility in: Epididymis
- Estrogen level after menopause: Reduced

- LSH is secreted by: Anterior pituitary
- Chvostek sign is seen in: Hypocalcemia
- Effect of calcitonin: Decreased serum calcium
- Somatostatin is secreted by: **Delta cells of pancreas**
- Hormone secreted by beta cells of pancreas: Insulin
- Calcium is absorbed maximally in: Proximal intestine
- Most potent stimulator of secretin release: Acidic chyme
- Site of absorption of iron: Duodenum
- Glucose transport occurs with: Sodium
- Major part of glomerular filtrate is absorbed in: PCT
- Decrease in pH shifts the oxygen dissociation curve to: Right
- Pneumotaxic centre is present in: Dorsal pons
- Pulmonary surfactant is produced by: Type II pneumocytes
- Amount of air breathed in or out during normal breathing is known as: Tidal volume
- Carbon di oxide is primarily transported in arterial blood as: Bicarbonates
- Third heart sound is due to: Ventricular filling
- QRS complex on ECG is due to: Ventricular depolarization
- Cardiac index is calculated as: cardiac output/ Body surface area
- Volume of blood ejected with each heart beat is known as: Stroke volume
- Blood pressure readings in thickened walled vessels & obesity: High
- Active sites of actin are covered by: Tropomyosin
- Intracellular fluid is rich in which cation: Potassium
- Site of ATP synthesis: Mitochondria
- Cell shape & motility is due to: Tubulin
- Size of action potential depends upon which ion: Sodium
- Repolarization of a nerve is due to which ion: Potassium
- Most abundant cation in extracellular fluid: Sodium
- Fertilization takes place in which part of fallopian tube: Ampulla
- Separation of 2nd polar body occurs at the time of: Fertilization
- Milk ejection is controlled by: Oxytocin
- Ovulation is due to surge of: LH
- Gas, responsible for respiratory drive: Carbon di oxide
- Temperature regulation is done by: Hypothalamus
- Action potential follows which law: All or none

- Platelets are stored at: 20-24 degree C
- Dreaming is commoner in which phase of sleep: REM
- Neurotransmitter depleted in Parkinson's disease: Dopamine
- Law explaining phantom limb: Law of projection
- Tract involved in Parkinson's disease: Nigro-striatal pathway
- Function of Kupffer cells in liver: Phagocytosis
- Chymo-trypsinogen is activated into chymotrypsin by: Trypsin
- Site of action of antidiuretic hormone/ ADH: Collecting duct & DCT
- Normal GFR is 125 ml/ min
- Reabsorption of water is maximum in: PCT
- Effect of parathormone on calcium levels: Increase in calcium levels
- Aortic valve closure marks the beginning of which phase of cardiac cycle: Phase of relaxation
- Calcitonin is secreted by: Parafollicular/ C cells of thyroid
- 1st heart sound is due to: Closure of AV valves
- Most useful for estimating total iron content of blood: Serum ferritin.
- D2O is used to measure the total body water.
- ECF can be measure with help of the Inulin.
- ICF can also be measure with help of D2O and Inulin.
- Factors affecting the total water of the body are fat, Age, obesity and sex.
- Osmolarity is the number of moles per litre of solution.
- Osmolality is the number of the osmoles per kg of solvent.
- Phagocytosis cell eating.
- Pinocytosis cell drinking.
- Clathrin mediated endocytosis (receptor mediated endocytosis).
- Transcytosis absorption by endocytosis and exocytosis.

- B lynch/Brace suture: uterus (PPH).
- Amniotic fluid mainly produced: fetus
- Blood loss in PPH: 500 ml (NVD). 1000 ml in LSCS
- 16 cells stage seen in merula.
- Another name of the Decidual shedoff: Decidual tree
- Triple screening test used in Down syndrome.
- Commonest congenital disease: heart
- Hela cells in Cervix.
- Clue cell in fallopian tube
- Length of the fallopian tube 12 cm
- Leukoplakia is the pre malignant lesion of the vulva.
- Fetal distress can be detected by scalp blood.
- Hegar sign commonly seen in 8 weeks
- Treatment of the asherman syndrome: D & C and IUCD.
- Multiple pregnancy commonly seen in: negros.
- Buddha sign seen: hydrops fetalis.
- Steroid effective in: IUGR
- Saffron colour meconium: **Post maturity.**
- Before onset of labour: PROM
- Post term labour: Anencephaly.
- Earliest sign of the IUD: **Robert's sign**
- Gas in great vessels seen in IUD.
- IUFD caused by PIH.
- Anencephaly: Face presentation.
- Alpha feto protein used to see the NTD.
- Common cause of the NTD: Folic acid.
- Classical cesarean section ca Cervix.
- Common type of episiotomy: RMLE.
- Common side effect of the magnesium sulphate: oligourea.
- Half-life of the syntonin: 3-4 minute.
- Best drug for the PPH: carboprost.
- Fetal requirement of iron: 300 mg.
- World population day: 11 july.
- World tobacco day: 31 may.

- World TB' day: 24 march.
- Breast feeding week: August.
- Main part of the umbilical cord: Wharton's jelly.
- Development of External genital: 8-12 weeks.
- Uterus weight at term: 1000 gm.
- Maximum level of beta HCG: 70 days of the pregnancy.
- Homologous organ to penis: clitoris.
- Master gland of the body: Pituitary gland.
- Bishop score related to labour.
- Mini pills commonly used in the lactating mother.
- Weight of the mother increased in pregnancy: 8-11 pounds.
- Placenta weight around 20% of the fetal weight.
- Aspermia after vasectomy 10-12 weeks.
- Prematurity is the common cause of the mortality of the twin baby.
- FSH secretion stimulated: LHRH
- 24 hours: LH surge.
- 10 weeks: should be diagnosed the anencephaly.
- Contraindication vaccine in pregnancy: TB
- Congenital cyst: Gartner's Cyst.
- Foetal serum: AFP level are highest
- Most rare cause of maternal mortility: Abortion.
- Most common cause of maternal mortility: hemorrhage.
- Perineal abscess common in the NVD delivery.
- DOC of the Cholera in pregnant lady: Azithromycin.
- Kocher's hemostatic forceps: umbilical cord.
- Commonest side effect of Cu-T: Bleeding.
- Hartman's sign: pregnancy.
- Prematurity: common cause of FM.
- Baby weight become double: 5 months/20 weeks.

Unani

- Ilm-e-Tib can be classified into Ilm-e-Hifze Sehat, Ilm-e-Ilaj.
- Ilm-e-Tib baitbar-e-Ilm can be classified into Tib-e-Ilmi/Nazri, Tib-e-Amli.
- Mozuat-e-Tib Insan, sehat,wa marz.
- Asbab has classified into Asbab-e-madiya, Asbab-e-faila, Asbab-e-Suriya and Asbab-e-Tamamiya.
- Asbab-e-Madiya is fundamental asbab for the sehat wa marz.
- Asbab-e-Faila has classified into Asbab-e-Sitta Zarooriya, Asbab Ghair zarooriya.
- Asbab-e-Sooriya has classified Mizaj, Quwa and Tarakeeb.
- Asbab-e-Tamimiya/ Ghaiya Afal-e-Badan Insani.
- Umoor-e-Tabiya are classified into Arkan, Mizaj, Ikhlat, Azaa, Arwah, Quwa and Afal.
- Ajza-e-Madiya Arkan, Ikhlat, Azaa and Arwah.
- Ajza-e-Sooriya Mizaj.
- Synonyms of the Arkan Ustokhusaat,Ajsam-e-Baseet.
- Single Anasir: 1. Bukhar 2. soil 3. Fire 4. Water 5.Air.
- Double Anasir: 6. Fire, Soil. 7.Soil, Water 8. Air, Soil.
- Three Anasir: 9. Fire, Air, Soil.
- Three Anasir 10. Air, Water, Soil (fire is the converted form of air).
- Three Anasir 11. Oil, Salt, and Kibreet.
- Four Anasir 12. Anasir-e-Arab (it is quoted by Arastu in Unani first).
- Five Anasir 13: Anasir-e-Arba + Sky.
- Anasir-e-Kaseera: Ashab-e-Khaleet.

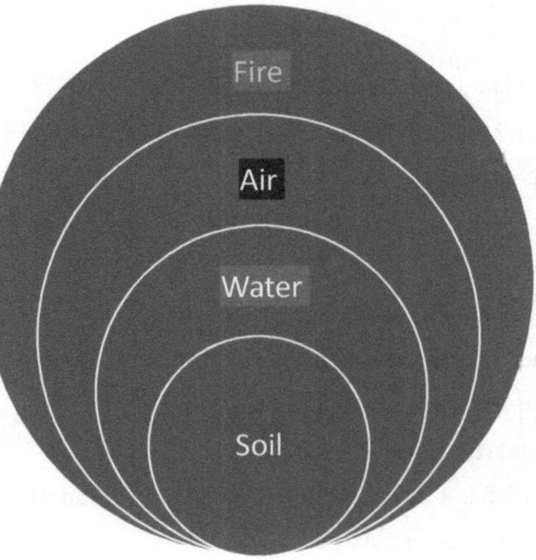

- Anasir-e-Arba: Accrding to the Kafiyat has been classified into Kafiyat-e-Faila and Kafiyat-e-Munfaila.
- Mizaj: Milna, Halool, Dakhool.
- Imtezaj-e-Sada: Like Combination of Water and Sugar.
- Imtezaj-e-Hakeeki: Like Roasting of the Sugar.
- Mizaj motadil and Mizaj-e-Ghair motadil.
- Mizaj-e-ghair motadil has 8 types.
- According to the Fakhruddin Razi Masihi. Mizaj of people living on Aqhleem-e-Charum is motadil.
- Human's Mizaj has deviated towards the Hararat and Ratoobat.
- According to the Ibn Sina. Mizaj of the people living on khat-e-istewa is motadil.
- Mizaj-e-Aza according to the kafiyat **Aza-e-Motadil, Aza-e-Haar, Aza-e-Barid, Aza-e-Ratab and Aza-e-Yabis.**
- Aza-e-Motadil: Skin < Skin of the hand < Palm (Raha) < Skin of the Fingers< First finger (Angasht Sababa).
- Aza-e-Haar: Heart (Qalb) < Liver (Jigar) < Muscle (Laham).
- Aza-e-Barid: Bone (Azam) < Ligaments (Rubat) < Nerves (Asab) < Brain (Dimagh).
- Aza-e-Ratab: Liquid fat (Sameen) < Riwaj < Muscle < brain (dimagh).
- Aza-e-Yabisa: Hair (Baal) < Bone (Haddi) < Ghazroof < Ligaments (Rubat).
- Hottest organ of the body is heart.
- Mizaj-e-Amar:
- Sin-e-Namu: Har Ratab

- Sin-e-Shabab: Har Yabis
- Sin-e-Kahulat: Barid Yabis
- Sin-e-Shekhookhat: Barid Ratab.
- Akhlat: Khilt-e-Dam, Khilt-e-Safra, Khilt-e-Balgham, Khilt-e-Sauda.
- Khilt-e-Dam divided into Dam-e-Tabai & Dam-e-Ghair Tabai.
- Features of the Dam-e-Tabai are Rooh-e-Mehlool, Surkh Rang, Bina Zaykha, Qiwam motadil and Shireen.
- Khit-e-Safra divided into Khilt-e-Safra-e-Tabai & Khilt-e-Safra-e-Ghair Tabai.
- Functions of the Khilt-e-Safra-e-Tabai: Munafae, Tarqeeqh-ud-dam, Taqhziya-e-Aza, Tahreek-e-Ama, Taqhseel-e-Ama, Halakat-e-Deedan, man-e-Ufoonat etc.
- Khilt-e-Safra Ghair tabai:
- Muhayya: It is the combination of Safra and Ghaleez Balgham.
- Murah: It is the combination of Safra and Raqeeq Balgham.
- Muthariqa: it occurs after combustion (Ahraq).
- Qurassi /Zanjari: Dark Green in colour.
- **Diseases of the Safra:**
- Jaundice (Yarqan-e-Asfar).
- Boil (Basoor-e-Safra)
- Stone of the liver (Hissat-e-Kabid).
- Cirrhosis of the liver (Siqhrul-e-Kabid)
- Nausea (Safrawi Qai)
- Loose Stools (Safrawi Ishal)
- Qulanj-e-Safrawi.
- Khilt-e-Balgham divided into Balgham-e-tabai and Balgham-e-ghair Tabai.
- **According to the taste Blagham has classified into:**
- Malah: Har Yabis
- Hamiz: Barid yabis
- Tufah: Barid Yabis
- Afaz: Barid
- Halu: Har Ratab
- **According to the Qiwam Blagham has classified into:**
- Mai: (Similar to water).
- Jassi: (Similar to Chuna)
- Kham: (Similar to Mukhat)

- Zujaji: (Similar to Glass)
- **According to the Bou Blagham has classified into:**
- Muntan: Boudar.
- **Functions of the Balgham:**
- Converted into blood, moisturize the Different organs, Nutrition to the organ.
- **Diseases of the Balgham:**
- Cold (Nazla)
- Tahabuj (Swelling)
- Nausea
- Loss stools (Ishal-e-Balghami)
- Bala-e-Asaliya.
- Vitiligo (Bars).
- Aza-e-Raisa has consider as Aza-e-Murakkaba (Compound).
- Shash has been consider as the Aza-e-Haiwaniya.
- Cause of the Warm-e-Sulb is Sauda.
- Best physician of the body is Tabiyat.
- Generally the Mizaj of the child move towards the Ratoobat.
- Ali Gilani has been proved in experiment the Mizaj are four type.
- Main organ of the Quwwat-e-Tabiya is Liver (Jigar).
- Main organ of the Quwwat-e-Haiwaniya is Heart (Qalb).
- Main organ of the Quwwat-e-Nafsaniya is Brain (Dimagh).
- Main organ of the Quwwat-e-Tanasulliya is Testis/Ovaries.
- According to the Ghiza, servant of the heart is Liver.
- Rooh is relates with lateef akhlat.
- Big amount of the rooh found in the vessels.
- According to the hazam-e-Arba (four type digestion) the hazam-e-kabdi is known as IInd digestion.
- Urine is the excreta of the hazam-e-Kabdi and Hazam-e-uzwi.
- Organ co relates in the Quwwat-e-Nafsaniya are brain, spinal cord, rooh-e-Nafsani.
- Quwwat-e-Faila works on the muscle (azlat).
- Parts of the Hazam-e-Maidi are Dehan (Saliva), Maida (Stomach), Ama (Colon) etc.
- Quwwat-e-Muqhiyrra Saniya works on the blood (Dam).
- Primary types of the Quwwat-e-Nafsaniya are two.

- Quwwat responsible for the production of the Mani (Semen) is known as Quwwat-e-Muwalida.
- Quwwat-e-Shamma relates with the Anf, (Nose).
- Centre of the Quwwat-e-Hafiza is hind brain (Muakhir dimagh).
- How many types of the afal-e-Hisiya are 4.
- Quwwat-e-Muwalida works on the ovaries/testis.
- Quwwat-e-Lamsa works on skin.
- Quwwat can be prove by the function.
- Balgham can be consider as the different form of the blood.

REFRENCES:

1. Moore's Clinically Oriented Anatomy 2021.

2. Gray's Anatomy for Students, 5th Edition 2023.

3. Netter Atlas of Human Anatomy: Classic Regional Approach, 8th Edition 2022.

4. Medical Physiology, 3rd Edition 2016.

5. Netter's Essential Systems-Based Anatomy, 1st Edition 2021.

6. Nolte's The Human Brain, 8th Edition 2020.

7. B. D chaurasia 8th edition 2022.

8. Essentials Of Medical Physiology Free Review Of Medical Physiology 2018.

9. Essentials Of Medical Physiology 2011.

10. Textbook Of Medical Physiology 2008.

Table of contents

FSC
www.fsc.org
MIX
Papier | Fördert
gute Waldnutzung
FSC® C083411

Kolibri 360 GmbH
Ferdinand-Jühlke-Straße 7
99095 Erfurt, Deutschland
produktsicherheit@kolibri360.de

Druck:
CPI Druckdienstleistungen GmbH
im Auftrag der
Kolibri 360 GmbH
Ferdinand-Jühlke-Str. 7
99095 Erfurt